<u>Losing the Baby Weight: A Quick Guide to a Fit Mind, Body, and Soul for Mothers</u> ©
By Meredith Majors

<u>An Organized Life Leads to Great Things</u>

Commitment to a goal will change your life. That is a true statement. Therefore, an organized life will help one focus on goals; and in this case: Losing the Baby Weight. Being a mother is a life-changing ordeal, and it can make or break some people. Don't let the challenge of motherhood make you doubt yourself: YOU CAN DO IT! All the while being in the best shape of your life! Being in good shape will only boost one's parental abilities. Furthermore, losing the baby weight is a commitment that will improve life in every way possible. Mothers want the best for their babies; and by getting organized, fit, and healthy: your baby will have the best mom possible!

Out of Sight, out of mind: De-Clutter

First things first: Get organized! After the commitment to lose the baby weight has been established, make a plan to get your life organized. Everyone is different, but the way I started organizing was by writing down a list. In other words, a plan of attack to get my unorganized, crazy life in gear. Don't worry because this cannot be accomplished in one day. It may take days or weeks, depending on the clutter and one's routine. You can do it though! It is possible, even though it may seem daunting.

Repeat to yourself as you clean: "Out of sight, out of mind." This is really true. When losing weight, it is imperative to have a tidy home. Clutter is not only bad for the baby, but it adds to the stress level of motherhood. Stress will not allow the body to get rid of the extra pounds. That is why we feel at peace when coming home to a clean house. **Therefore, one of the consistent goals every day is to find inner peace through the result of a tidy home.**

There are many ways to organize the clutter. Everything in one's home should have a place; this way you know exactly where to find it. Also, it will become easier and easier to clean every day when things have their place in the home. Routine and order are wonderful for peace of mind. Don't get me wrong, I'm not saying to become obsessive compulsive, but finding balance is the name of the game.

If you are having trouble organizing, look into stores that specialize in organization. Or find inspirational photos online or in magazines. Closets can be transformed into a beautiful cache of your stuff. Your home can look like it deserves to be showcased in Home & Gardens. You just need a plan and the execution of said plan to get you there.

I now enjoy looking at pictures of organized homes and closets. Also known as organization porn to some. These photos of tidiness inspire me to keep working hard, because everything starts with getting organized. And by the way, be sure to not throw random items into a junk drawer or stuff things into a closet without any sort of order whatsoever. Out of sight, out of mind is true but only works if it is done the right way. However, don't beat yourself up if it takes time to get it all done the right way. Just as long as it gets done. Just as a baby takes nine months to develop, it will take you baby steps to get organized; so enjoy the process and don't get overwhelmed.

A suggestion on where to start: Clean out your purse and your wallet. Take everything out, and place on a table or floor. Get rid of garbage and clutter. A small make-up bag is useful for lipstick and compact powder. Take a baby wipe or warm wet cloth and clean the inside and outside of your purse. I sometimes vacuum it out then clean it. Whatever you decide to do, clean and organize the best you can. It will serve you well, I promise!

If you can never find anything in your purse, consider getting a smaller one; possibly one with an organizer built in. With the baby, you will have a diaper bag; therefore, a big bulky purse may not be suitable for the time being. Perhaps find a purse and diaper bag in one? As long as you find something that works for you and stick with it. Make your life as efficient as possible. It will make you smile to have an organized purse and wallet; not to mention clean inside and out! Then move on to your car, then your closet, then the kitchen, and so on and so forth; until everything in your life is organized to the T (for Tidy.)

One last suggestion: if something is not being used or useful, providing some sort of joy or purpose, then get rid of it! Life is so much better when clutter is gone! Out of sight, out of mind.

Meditation and Prayer

Meditation and prayer are very important as well, and I suggest making time for this daily. Even when you're organizing, these mental exercises will only help you focus on the task at hand. The reason these are listed second is because I truly believe that when your life is organized, the clarity and practice of meditation and prayer is infinitely more refined.

There are many ways to accomplish mental focus, and that is the purpose of Meditation and Prayer. Therefore, whatever brings you to a calm, peaceful state of mind then do that exercise. Meditation can be stretching and breathing exercises. Sitting comfortably on the floor, with eyes closed, and deep breath in and out. Then repeat for 10-15 minutes, possibly longer.

Yoga is an excellent practice for a combination of meditation and strength training (more about yoga in *Body & Fitness*). Reading is also a great way to relax and focus. Some read the bible and spend time praying each day. No matter if you're religious or not, the key to success is focusing on the things you desire and keeping the main goal locked in your mind daily which is: Losing the Baby Weight.

Communication

Great leaders lead with their hearts, and are not afraid to communicate with their team for help. As a mother, you're a leader and you cannot expect to do everything by yourself. Therefore, it is important to communicate with family and friends when you need a day to yourself; or need assistance. A mental health day at the spa. Or a trip to the mall for fun. Request that your significant other watch the baby while you catch up on some much needed rest. People in your life are there for you, as you are for them. Learning to communicate your needs with others can lead to greater bonds and relationships in the long run. Not to mention, it can lead to a more rested, vibrant, happy, supported version of yourself every day.

It is perfectly okay to ask for help, even if you need to vent about your stresses. As a mother, I thought I could handle all my problems myself, and I now wish I would have reached out more to friends and family for assistance. I currently reach out for help daily, and I am so much happier! A team keeps your mind balanced and has your back when issues pop up. Feeling alone, and trying to do too much on your own, is a huge stress that can be remedied by simply communicating with the people you trust.

Some people may choose to talk to their pastor, counselor, or therapist for guidance as well. Communicating is extremely important, especially when committing to a goal of losing weight and changing your entire life's routine to make it happen. It is imperative to not allow scheduling issues to interfere with your progress. Therefore, make a plan, communicate with your team (friends, family, and community), and make no excuses getting things done.

For example, if you need an hour to workout, before starting your day, and your spouse cannot help: have a backup team member to call. If they're busy, have a 3rd member ready on speed dial. Make it happen, because you need help in order to accomplish your goals. Do not be afraid to communicate with your loved ones, it will only serve to help you.

Community and Family

It is normal for women to want to stay home and workout; especially after having a baby. However, getting out of the house is a must; unless you are really good at holding yourself accountable, and most of us are just not. Therefore, get involved with your community activities, such as running for a specific cause. Or joining a fitness group- whether it be yoga, running, or a gym membership- will hold you accountable, and will be a part of your scheduled routine. It is also imperative to have another support system in your journey to weight loss; as well as fun! Get a trusted friend to go with you to yoga once or twice a week. Workout with your significant other once a week. The whole point is to get out of the house, get involved with your community, and make it fun and enjoyable.

You may be thinking: *How do I have time to do all this stuff?* You can achieve anything with determination, a positive spirit, a support system, and a plan of action. This is why it is crucial to be organized, and have a schedule: daily, monthly, and yearly. You can accomplish so much when you have a plan, and then execute it the best way possible. No one starts college without a syllabus, class schedule, and reading materials. Everything is in place for a reason, and set up for success. This is why I cover organization first, and foremost, because it leads us to a triumphant conclusion to our goals. In this case: Losing the Baby Weight. However, once you lose the baby weight, keeping a schedule and staying organized will also keep the pounds off. And organization skills will accompany you to succeeding at any goal you set forth from here on out!

When I was a kid, my mom would go for a 3 mile run after she got home from work. I would accompany her by riding my bike. I remember enjoying one on one time with my mom, and we got our exercise for the day: win win for both of us! Getting healthy starts with commitment, but making it fun by spending time with friends and family is a bonus!

<u>Nutrition is Key</u>

Prior to beginning any new diet regime, please consult with your doctor, and be weary of your recommended daily caloric intake. Please note: If you are breastfeeding, your caloric intake will be higher per your doctor's specified advice.

Similar to a car, our bodies need fuel; and the kind of fuel we put in our tanks gives us different results in performance. I'm not a mechanic, but I have rescued a few friends on the side of the road, due to their cars running out of gas or breaking down etc. Cars and fuel works as a metaphor, because this is all true of our human bodies as well. If we eat junk, our bodies turn into junk, and our minds cannot focus; which creates an endless cycle of tiredness and no progression whatsoever. Our bodies cannot perform without the proper nutrition; aka fuel.

We must return to basic, healthy food groups; and most importantly- repeat after me: ADDED SUGAR IS EVIL AND TOXIC. Jumping back to the car metaphor: Do you know what happens if someone pours a bag of sugar in your car's gas tank? Answer: your car would die, and never run again. This is true, just ask your mechanic. Added Sugar will do the same to our human bodies as it does to our cars: kills our performance and potential. So sorry if that scares you, but it is the truth. On that note, let's start off nutrition with the most important lesson in Losing the Baby Weight: ADDED SUGAR IS EVIL AND TOXIC.

Added Sugar is Evil and Toxic

Before I begin on how Added Sugar is evil and toxic, please note that I am speaking of many types of Added Sugar: Cane Sugar, Brown Sugar, Sugar in the Raw, High Fructose Corn Syrup, Maple Syrup, Honey, Agave Nectar, Organic Sugar, Coconut Sugar, etc etc etc. The sugary sweetness has many names, but all mean the same thing; and in excess it turns toxic in our bodies. Anything sweet that one has to add into their food or drink is "Added Sugar." Anything plant derived, such as fruit, is NOT considered "Added Sugar." Also note that cow's milk sugar is not Added Sugar either. However, sweetened Almond Milk has Added Sugar. Don't worry though: Almond Milk has an unsweetened version to enjoy! Just keep an eye on "Sugar" in the listed ingredients. (Ingredients: Almonds, Water, Sugar ← "Added Sugar.")

Now keep in mind: that all the fake sugars, such as splenda, equal, and sweet n low etc are even more harmful to your body. Fake sugars are in the category of "Added Sugars" as well. More to come on added sugar as we go, but let me take a few steps back to explain in more detail.

I am from a small city in the Southern United States, which is all about eating Added Sugar and anything fried. Not to mention, the South is known to be the fattest in America. Therefore, I was addicted to sugar for most of my life. My weight would always fluctuate, and I was tired every day. Now that I am no longer addicted to Added Sugar, my life has changed for the absolute best. My weight no longer fluctuates, I am the smallest I've ever been, and I have so much energy with no caffeine in my diet.

I remember reading fitness authors say similar things, and it would just make me mad. I would defend my Added Sugar to the brutal end! I thought it was all about calories in and calories out; but I was wrong. By becoming a personal fitness trainer with a certification in

6

Wellness and Nutrition; as well as a degree in Anatomy and Physiology- I set out to discover the truth and finally get *truly* healthy.

I do know and understand the human body; but I defended Added Sugar for years- never again, though; because I've seen my life on the other side of this evil toxic addiction. Added Sugar has been a topic of discussion in the health field for decades- since the 1950s, actually. Therefore, I recommend watching a documentary film that changed my life (for the better). The documentary is called: *Sugar Coated*, and it is available on Netflix or On Demand. Google it, and watch it tonight! After watching this documentary, within the next 2 weeks, I lost 10 pounds! I'm talking about the 10 hardest pounds to lose. The extra fluff, which always sat on top of my muscles, was gone! And I was still breastfeeding, eating all the time- just without the Added Sugar! Everything changed for me after watching that film.

Have you ever wondered why we crave Added Sugar? It's because Added Sugar is so concentrated and processed that are bodies cannot break it down properly. Therefore, it gives us this high euphoric feeling, before crashing into moodiness, followed by an exhausted feeling. We've all heard of the sugar crash. This kind of reaction is not healthy; and is the bodies' way of telling us something bad is going on. I experienced withdrawals when I quit Added Sugar, just like a heroin addict: horrible headaches, thirsty all the time, and I was very moody. It was truly an eye-opening experience. However, once the withdrawals ceased, I felt better than ever before. And I was truly happy!

~Natural Sugar versus Added Sugar~

Fruits, veggies, and other plant derived foods have natural sugar; this is different than "Added Sugar." Natural sugars are easily broken down by the body, but only as nature intended: in small doses. Some would say Cane Sugar is natural, but let me explain an important fact as to why it boils down to how things are processed. For instance, granulated sugar is processed from a plant, called Sugar Cane. Most people know this, but not many people consider how much Sugar Cane Plant it takes to make 1 pound of granulated sugar. Do you know how granulated sugar is processed? Below is an illustration diagram on how the sugar cane plant is processed into granulated sugar.

FROM CANE SUGAR TO GRANULATED SUGAR

Crazy, isn't it? Even if they stopped at Raw Sugar, the 6th step in the process, and skipped so much of the other chemical break-down, our bodies are not built to consume so many Sugar Cane Plants in one sitting. In other words, let's break it down to simple sugar math.

~Simple Sugar Math~

1. An average sugarcane stalk weighs about 3 pounds (1.3 kilograms) and is 85% juice. How many pounds of juice will an average stalk produce?

Answer: 2.6 pounds (1.1 kilograms) of juice.

2. The juice squeezed out of a sugarcane stalk is about 11% sugar by weight. How many pounds of sugar can be produced from one stalk?

8

Answer: An average stalk contains about 0.3 pounds (0.12 kilograms) of sugar.

3. How many stalks of sugarcane will it take to produce a 5-pound bag of sugar?

Answer: 16.67 canes are needed to make 5 pounds of granulated sugar. (Roughly 50 pounds of sugarcane stalks to make 5 pounds of granulated sugar.)

In 2015, the average American consumed 66.6 pounds of refined sugar, 62 pounds of corn-derived sweeteners, 1.5 pounds of honey and edible syrups, for a total caloric-sweetener annual consumption of 154.8 pounds. Yikes! All stats were found on FAITC.org (US Agriculture School Statistics.)

I know it is hard to follow because we are talking about sugar here! Let me break it down another way, because one truly needs to understand this in order to succeed in losing the baby weight. How would you feel after eating 1 orange versus 10 oranges? I think most people would have a tummy ache if they consumed 10 oranges in one sitting. Sugar Cane Stalk is a plant as well; therefore, if we look at it unprocessed, in its original state, and tried to eat it -one would look at Added Sugar very differently.

Coca cola that is made from cane sugar (not corn sugar) has roughly 1 processed stalk of sugar cane worth of Added Sugar. It's tough to compute why this is so horrible, but follow me on this important mindset change. Going back to the oranges, it is not nature's intention for us to eat 10 oranges in one sitting; just as it is not natural for us to eat a 3 pound stalk of Sugar Cane.

If you ever ate honeysuckle as a kid, it would take hundreds of honeysuckle flowers to make a teaspoon of juice. Same with Sugar Cane: only 11% of the juice extracted from the 3 pound stalk is processed into granulated sugar (roughly 39 grams or 10 teaspoons of Added Sugar.)

Our bodies can break down small doses of Added Sugar in a day, but no more than 20 grams before our liver gets overloaded (like a traffic jam on the freeway.) 20 grams is not very much compared to how much a normal person consumes of Added Sugar. To put in perspective, an average person consumes 76 grams of added sugar per day.

Before I realized how damaging Added Sugar was to my body, I consumed at least 100 grams of added sugar a day. I have been an athlete my whole life, and have always worked out; but I still had trouble with my weight. I drank at least 2 cans of cola per day, ate granola bars, and sweet cereals etc. etc. etc. Not to mention, my teeth had cavities every time I went to the dentist. Added Sugar is in so much food that it is no wonder so many struggle with it.

Taming Added Sugar in your diet will create an amazing change in your body and life; this change alone will do wonders! Okay, so if you want to truly get healthy and feel better than you've ever felt before: you need to follow this *Back to the Basics* guide in nutrition. It is eating like nature intended, and your plate will always be filled with yummy food. If you love to eat, then you will love getting *Back to the Basics*! Follow along with me in the next section for easy nutrition guidelines, on how to tame Added Sugar, and to start feeling great again! I know it sounds difficult, but it isn't; and it will be a big change for the better. **You Can Do It! And You are Worth It!**

Back to the Basics: Classic Food Pyramid

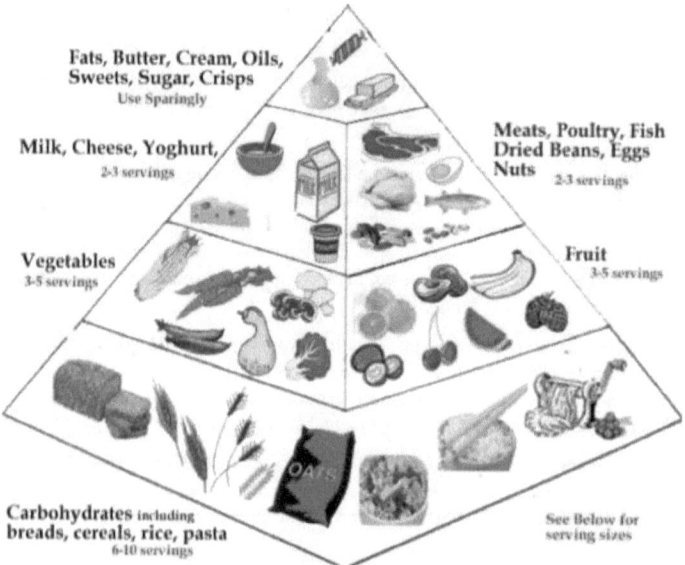

Food Pyramid

The food pyramid was developed by the U.S. Department of Agriculture (USDA) as a nutrition guide for healthy persons over the age of two years. The guide stresses eating a wide variety of foods from the five major food groups while minimizing the intake of fats and Added Sugars. The daily quantity of foods from each group is represented by the triangular shape. The pyramid is composed of four levels. The tip represents fats and sweets, the second level emphasizes foods primarily from animals (milk and meat groups), the third level emphasizes foods from plants (vegetable and fruit groups), and the bottom level emphasizes foods from grains (breads, cereals, and rice).

The recommended servings of each food group are expressed in ranges so that the pyramid can fit most members of a household. The number of servings chosen from each food group is based upon the number of calories a person needs. A **calorie** is the amount of **energy** obtained from food. Most persons should always have at least the lowest number of servings for each group. In general, the low to middle numbers of servings are appropriate for most women and the middle to upper numbers of servings are appropriate for most men.

Fats, Oils, and Sweets

Fats, oils, and sweets are at the very top of the pyramid because these foods should be used sparingly. In general, these foods provide only calories, little else nutritionally. Persons should choose lower fat foods from each group, reduce the use of fats (such as butter) and sugars (such as jelly) at the table, and reduce the intake of sweet foods (soda, candy, etc.).

Fats should not contribute more than 30% of a persons' daily calories. To determine the number of grams of fat that contributes 30% of the calories multiply the total day's calories by 0.30 and divide by 9. For example, a 2,200 calorie diet should contain no more than 2.5 oz (73 g) of fat.

Milk, Yogurt, and Cheese

The food pyramid recommends two to three servings of milk products daily. Women who are pregnant or breast feeding, teenagers, and adults up to the age of 24 years need three servings daily. Milk products are the best food source of calcium and also provide protein, minerals, and vitamins. A serving size is one cup of milk or yogurt, 2 oz (56 g) of processed cheese, or 1.5 oz (43 g) of natural cheese. There are lactose free options as well.

Meat, poultry, fish, dry beans, eggs, and nuts

The food pyramid recommends eating two to three servings (or 5-7 oz [142-198 g] of meat) from this group. Meat, fish, and poultry provide protein, iron, zinc, and B vitamins. Eggs, nuts, and dry beans supply protein, vitamins, and minerals. To help determine the serving size of meats, an average hamburger is about 3 oz. One half a cup of cooked dry beans, 2 tbsp of peanut butter, one egg, or one third a cup of nuts are all equivalent to 1 oz (28 g) of meat.

Lean meats and poultry should be chosen to reduce the intake of fat and cholesterol. Lean meats include: sir-loin steak, pork tenderloin, veal (except ground), lamb leg, chicken and turkey (without skin), and most fish. The intake of nuts and seeds, which contain large amounts of fat, should be reduced.

Vegetable

The food guide pyramid recommends eating three to five servings of vegetables each day. Vegetables provide vitamins, minerals, and fiber, and are low in fat. A serving size of vegetable is 1 cup of raw salad greens, one half a cup of other cooked or raw vegetables, or three quarters of a cup of vegetable juice. Limit the use of toppings or spreads (butter, salad dressing, mayonnaise, etc.) because they add fat and Added Sugar calories.

The food pyramid recommends eating a variety of vegetables because different classes of vegetables provide different nutrients. Vegetables classes include: dark green leafy (broccoli, spinach, romaine lettuce, etc.), deep yellow (sweet potatoes, carrots, etc.), starchy (corn, potatoes, peas, etc.), legumes (kidney beans, chickpeas, etc.), and others (tomatoes, lettuce, onions, green beans, etc.). The vegetable subgroups dark green leafy and legume should be chosen often because they contain more nutrients than other vegetables. Also, legumes can substitute for meat.

Fruit

The food guide pyramid recommends two to four servings of fruit daily. Fruits provide vitamin A, vitamin C, and potassium and are low in fat. A serving size of fruit is three quarters of a cup of fruit juice, one half a cup of cooked, chopped, or canned fruit, or one medium sized banana, orange, or apple.

The food pyramid recommends choosing fresh fruits, 100% fruit juices, and canned, frozen, or dried fruits. Intake of fruits that are frozen or canned in heavy syrup should be limited. Whole fruits are preferred because of their high fiber content. Melon, citrus, and berries contain high levels of vitamin C and should be chosen frequently. Juices that are called punch, -ade, or drink often contain considerable Added Sugar and only a small amount of fruit juice.

Bread, cereal, rice, and pasta

With 6-11 servings daily, this food group is the largest group, hence the bottom position on the pyramid. This group provides complex carbohydrates (starches), which are long chains of sugars, as well as vitamins, minerals, and fiber. Carbohydrates are the gasoline for the body's many energy-requiring systems (good sugars). A serving size from this group is one slice of bread, 1 oz (27 g) of cold cereal, or one half a cup of pasta, rice, or cooked cereal.

Complex carbohydrates in and of themselves are not fattening, it is the spreads and sauces used with these foods that add the most calories. For the most nutrition, foods prepared from whole grains (whole wheat bread or whole grain cereals for instance) with little added fat and/or sugar should be chosen. The intake of high fat and/or high sugar baked goods (cakes, cookies, croissants, etc.) and the use of spreads (butter, jelly, etc.) should be reduced.

**Food Pyramid Information and Recommendations provided by Encyclopedia.com

As a mom, the best nutrition for our baby is a priority; so why not have the same standard for ourselves? When I was breastfeeding, everything I ate was going to my baby; therefore, my mindset suddenly became super protective of how I consumed food. I no longer consumed Added Sugar for my go to fix, and I didn't drink caffeine. I was committed to eating healthy because of my sweet baby girl, and without her- I probably would still be addicted to sugar and struggling every day. Therefore, I am so grateful to be a mother; and I hope going *Back to the Basics: Food Pyramid* will bring you the same joy it has brought to me and my family.

The Food Pyramid is filled with wonderful, yummy foods, and is so easy to follow. The biggest change will be cutting back on the Added Sugar and Fats from your diet. Remember this means fake sugar as well. There has been much discussion on Stevia, because it is made from a plant; but I would suggest to use any Added Sugar (fake or not) sparingly. My opinion is to stop consuming fake sugar all together, it would be the best choice for your body.

Please note: you will need to start examining labels and ingredients. For example, let's examine a yummy bowl of cereal. Cereals used to be my favorite snack food. I would eat cocoa puffs, lucky charms, frosted flakes, and any sugary sweet cereal I could get my hands on. Oh boy, do they have a lot of Added Sugar! Remember no more than 20 grams of added sugar a day (and if you can go lower the better.) I still eat cereal every day but I found a clever way to beat the addiction of Added Sugar; and still keep to the Food Pyramid Guide for Nutrition.

Following along with our trusty Food Pyramid: we need to consume 6-10 servings of Carbohydrates a day; this includes breads, cereals, pasta, and rice. Milk is also on the Food Pyramid with 2-3 servings per day, and has 9-12 grams of Natural Sugar, so it doesn't count in the "Added Sugar" bad list. Therefore, one way to enjoy yummy cereal (by following the Food Pyramid) is to choose Corn Flakes and cut up bananas and raspberries on top with your milk. Corn Flakes has 2 grams of added sugar, but fruit sugars are natural so the bananas and raspberries don't count (keep in mind that fruit servings are 3-5 servings per day.) One fruit serving would be equal to one banana. Therefore, a half a banana and a handful of raspberries would be one serving of fruit on your cereal.

I drink Unsweetened Almond Milk because I like it, and I am Lactose Intolerant; but there is no added sugar and only 30 calories per cup. Score! I know it seems like a great deal to follow, but once you go *Back to the Basics: Food Pyramid* and remember to keep count of your Added Sugar -it will get easier. Eating fruits, veggies, meats, carbs, cheeses and keeping the added sugar, and oils on watch, you will enjoy eating again- because you will get to eat so much!

Keep an eye on added sugar in breads, pastas, and other carbohydrate foods. I eat "Butter Bread" from Nature's Own, because it only has 1 added sugar gram per slice. I enjoy whipped cream cheese on my bread, but I make sure to not buy the added sugar cream cheeses. Instead, I add just cinnamon on top of the spread for added flavor and no added sugar.

Also, be watchful of bars: there's a whole isle of bars at the grocery store. Oh boy, most granola bars and protein bars have tons of Added Sugar. However, if you want to waste most of your allotted added sugar grams on a small bar then, by all means, do it. Though, I would suggest to stick to fruits for the sweet fix that nature intended for our bodies. Eating a beautiful honeycrisp apple will take many delicious bites, and is only around 60-70 calories (depending the size.) A protein bar has added sugar or fake sugar, and is normally more than 150 calories. Not to mention, 3-4 bites is over pretty quickly with not the same satiating qualities as an apple.

Understanding Calories Burned from Breast Feeding

If you're still breastfeeding, this section is important for staying focused on calories in versus calories out; and understanding how to calculate calories burned from breastfeeding. When I began breastfeeding, I was told by nurses, family, and friends that breastfeeding burns a gazillion calories. Well, vagueness like this was not going to help me stay on track with my nutrition; so I set out to make sure I understood numbers for my daughter's health and my own. I was always hungry while breastfeeding. My daughter breastfed often, and I had to eat more meals to keep up with her intake.

It is imperative not to starve or deprive yourself for the goal of losing weight; especially when supplying breast milk for your baby. However, it is important to understand how all of the breastfed calories are calculated -so you can prepare and plan for your day of meals.

It gets tricky on how to measure how much milk your baby gets through breastfeeding; but pumping actually has its advantages! By pumping both breasts, you can measure exactly how many ounces you are producing. Therefore, it's very easy to calculate your caloric output of milk.

- **Each ounce of breast milk has 20 calories. Therefore, 30 ounces per day would equal 600 calories burned. (20 calories x 30 ounces of milk= 600 calories burned.)**

Now to be even more exact, we need to calculate the production efficiency, or the energy used to produce the milk, which is 80% of the milk (energy) produced. So here is the formula to get the total calories burned from the milk you produce and the energy it takes to produce the milk.

- **Therefore, 30 ounces of milk per day x 20 calories = 600 calories burned divided by 0.8 production efficiency = 750 total calories burned.**

Now if you're not an exclusive pumper, and want to determine how much milk your baby is consuming, there are a few options. By using a baby weight scale, weigh your baby before and after every feeding. You can buy these scales online at Amazon. Subtract the before weight from the after-feeding weight to determine how much milk was consumed. At the end of the day, take the total of milk consumed and multiply by 20 then divide by 0.8. Another option is to pump and bottle feed your baby within a 24 hour period. Then calculate the total amount of ounces consumed by 20 then divide by 0.8. Understanding calories in and calories out will help in the long run for losing the baby weight, and keeping it off.

Water, Water, Water, and More Water

Our bodies are made up of mostly water; therefore, we must stay hydrated constantly to maintain top performance potential. We've all heard before that the standard is 8 glasses of water intake for adults. I don't know about you but, for me, it was hard to accomplish this task of drinking water most days. I had my reusable water bottle, but it seemed impossible to drink so much water.

Once I stopped drinking so many sugary drinks, drinking water became second nature to me. Drinking tons of water also helps us to not over eat. Throughout my day, I chug water. Yes, I said "chug." I say this because it is the only way, I have found, to get all the required water for the day. By chugging the water, it also increases your metabolism to help burn more calories for the day. Score! Therefore, this is only my suggestion to succeed at drinking H2O; but you may find some other method that works better for you. And, by all means, whatever works –do it!

I, however, get up in the morning and immediately chug water. That's the first thing I do, because it's great to flush your system after a nights rest. I have a cup that measures exactly 8 ounces that I keep next to the kitchen sink. I chug two 8 ounce glasses of water. Then I have my breakfast; and after I've eaten, I chug 2 more 8 ounce glasses of water. I do this water routine for every meal. Whenever I'm in the kitchen, I try to chug water as well. All throughout the day. Most days, I can chug up to 100 ounces of water; and if I work out -as much as 120 ounces.

If you are breastfeeding, it is imperative to consume more water than the suggested eight 8 ounce glasses. The body works better when its hydrated, and your digestive system will thank you for the extra fluids. In the past, I have also used a gallon jug to monitor my water intake. I would fill up the gallon jug with water, and my goal was to drink the entire thing within 24 hours. As I said before, whatever works for you – do it! Just be sure to drink <u>at least</u> ten 8 ounce glasses of water a day = 80 ounces of beautiful H2O.

Sample Diets and Back-to-Basic Recipes
An example of my diet for one day is below.

Breakfast: Consists of 2/ 8oz glasses of water (chug chug) before I eat anything. Then I have a banana or cut of fruit salad in a small bowl. I then chug another 2/ 8 oz glasses of water. I feed my baby. Then I eat a hard-boiled egg with salt and pepper. I then eat 2 pieces of Nature's Own Butter Bread with whipped cream cheese and cinnamon (I usually share with my daughter). I then make hot herbal tea, always decaf.

Snack: Consists of downing 2/ 8oz glasses of water before eating. Serving of Organic Blue Corn Chips, with serving of hummus dip and a pickle spear. (Servings sizes are listed on labels.) And a hard-boiled egg with salt and pepper.

Lunch: Chugging 2/ 8oz glasses of water before eating. Large green-leafy salad with grilled salmon steak or chicken. Kraft Greek Salad Dressing (Serving size). Or sometimes I use lemon juice, salt, and pepper as my dressing. A dressing that is no more than 1 gram of sugar is what I aim for. Add feta cheese and an olive. 5-7 carrots and other veggies. Handful of crackers or small baguette. I end the meal chugging 2/ 8oz glasses of water. If I'm still hungry (not usually) I will eat a small baked potato with a serving size of butter.

Snack: Chugging 2/ 8oz glasses of water. Corn Flakes (1-2 serving size) with serving of unsweetened almond milk. I sometimes add fruit (raspberries and banana) on top.

Dinner: Yep, you guessed it I chug 2/ 8oz glasses of water before eating. Hamburger steak cooked with shallots, garlic, garlic powder, sea salt, and pepper. Steamed broccoli, and a baked sweet potato with a serving of butter (maybe cinnamon). Last 2/ 8 oz glasses of water. Then I eat an apple or small fruit salad. I love herbal tea at night too.

I hope my sample diet helps you understand a little better of the concept. Serving sizes are important, as well as sticking to the Basic Food Pyramid. If you cheat, you're only cheating yourself and your fitness goals. Not to mention, if you're breastfeeding- everything goes to your baby; so why not give your baby the best! Nutrition is everything! You CAN and WILL do it!!

**Below are sample diets for optimal results. Consult your doctor with any questions or for specific post-partum diet requirements. Also, do not consume foods in which you or your baby has a known allergy.

Most importantly: keep count of your added sugar grams (Only 20 grams per day, try to do less.) Added Sugar is in everything: dressings, yogurt, bars, drinks, breads, and more. Just remember milk and fruits have natural sugars, so look at the ingredients for added sugar or high fructose corn syrup (there are many names for sugar.) Sugar will be listed under ingredients; for example: milk, **cane sugar**, **high fructose corn syrup**, berries (natural sugar), etc. If the ingredients.

JILLIAN MICHAELS RIPPED IN 30

Find the recipes, nutritional information and cooking instructions for each of the meals below in the accompanying recipe file. The recipes are organized alphabetically by meal.

30 DAY MEAL PLAN

	Breakfast	Lunch	Snack	Dinner
Day 1	2 Eggs and Toast	Turkey and Avocado Wrap	Apple Berry Banana Smoothie	Turkey Kebabs
Day 2	Yogurt, Berries and Almonds	Grilled Sirloin Salad	Almonds and an Orange	Chicken Satay
Day 3	Waffles and Bananas	Mexican Pizza	Protein Bar	Black Bean Chili
Day 4	Ezekiel English Muffin or Toast with Almond Butter	Hummus and Vegetable Pita	Turkey Jerky	Roasted Salmon
Day 5	Oatmeal with Apples and Pecans	Seared Tuna Salad	Hard-Boiled Egg With an Apple	BBQ Chicken and Black Bean Burrito
Day 6	Egg White Breakfast Wrap	Chickpea Burgers	Hummus and Veggies	Honey-Lemon Marinated Chicken Breasts
Day 7	Cheerios with a Banana or Berries	Subway Veggie Delite	Popchips and Cottage Cheese	Zesty Shrimp Veracruzana
Day 8	Cottage Cheese and Pineapple	Salmon and Blueberry Salad	Baked Corn Chips and Salsa	Mediterranean Pizza
Day 9	Bagel and Cream Cheese	Chicken Salad With Avocado and Mango	Sunflower Seeds and Watermelon	Mahi Mahi Tacos
Day 10	Baked Sweet Potato and Sausage	Grilled Veggie Salad	Mozzarella Cheese and a Pear	Nut-Encrusted Chicken Breasts

To save ink in your printer please print this in black and white.

*Product can be found at www.jillianmichaels.com/shop and fine retailers.

WANT EVEN MORE WAYS TO GET RIPPED?

Get a **FREE 30 DAY** membership to Jillian's online program at
www.jillianmichaels.com/ripped30dvd

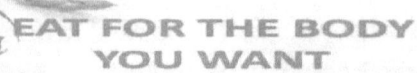

EAT FOR THE BODY YOU WANT
LOSE WEIGHT + BURN FAT

HEALTHY. SIMPLE. DELICIOUS.
MEAL PLAN DAY 1

BREAKFAST		7:00 AM
2	Eggs (any style)	
2 cups	Spinach	
2	Bell peppers	
1/4	Avocado	
1/2	Grapefruit	

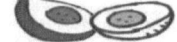
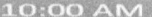

SNACK		10:00 AM
2 tbsps	Peanut butter	
1	Apple	

LUNCH		1:00 PM
4 oz	Chicken breask without skin	
1/2 cup	Cooked quinoa	
1 cup	Asparagus	
1 cup	Broccoli	
1/2 oz	Walnuts	

SNACK		4:00 PM
1 oz	Almonds	
1/2 cup	Berries	

DINNER		7:00 PM
4 oz	Grilled salmon	
2 cups	Arugula	
1 cup	Cherry tomatoes	
1/2 cup	Brown rice	
1/2 oz	Vinaigrette dressing	

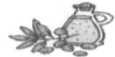

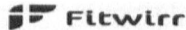

Fitwirr

18

STRAWBERRY BANANA LACTATION SMOOTHIE

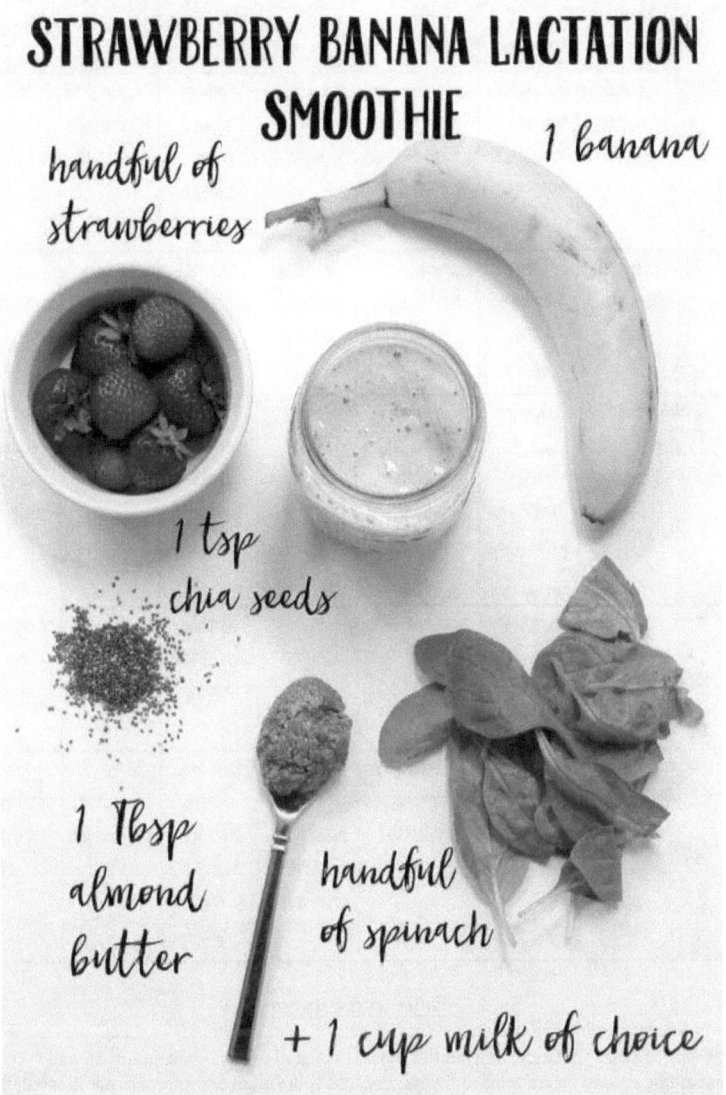

handful of strawberries

1 banana

1 tsp chia seeds

1 Tbsp almond butter

handful of spinach

+ 1 cup milk of choice

	Monday	Tuesday	Wednesday	Thursday	Friday	Saturday	Sunday
Breakfast	2 egg omelette w/tomatoes & avocado	Protein shake w/ strawberries	scrambled eggs, bacon, sauteed spinach, tomatoes	Protein shake w/ strawberries	Sausage topped w/ mozzarella & tomatoes	2 egg omelette w/tomatoes & avocado	Protein shake w/ strawberries
Snack 1	cucumber slices w/ ranch dressing	Cherry Tomatoes	cucumber slices w/ ranch dressing	Bell pepper slices w/ dressing	Celery w/ cream cheese	Bell pepper slices w/ dressing	Celery w/ cream cheese
Lunch	chicken quarter (w/skin) lettuce & Tomatoes	Burger (no bun) w/ cheese, avocado & tomato salad	Protein shake w/ strawberries & banana	Tuna with avocado, cucumber & tomato salad	lettuce wrapped chicken breast,fresh guacamole & salsa	Burger on chopped salad	Tuna with avocado, cucumber & tomato salad
Snack 2	Celery w/ cream cheese	cucumber slices w/ ranch dressing	bell pepper slices w/ dressing	cherry tomatoes	cucumber slices w/ ranch dressing	cherry tomatoes	bell pepper slices w/ dressing
Dinner	Pork tenderloin, sauteed spinach, grilled squash	Sirloin steak, sauteed bok choy, mixed green salad	Chicken, steamed broccoli, chopped spinach salad	Grilled burger w/ cheddar, baked sweet potato fries, mixed greens	Chicken breast, steamed broccoli & cauliflower, mixed green salad	Bangers & sweet potato mash, sauteed spinach	Steak, asparagus, mixed green salad

Body and Fitness

Once your mind and life are free of clutter, and your nutrition is in check, exercise and fitness will be easier and more of a central focus. I covered organization, nutrition, and understanding caloric intake prior to fitness: because if the mind and spirit are not focused, then ultimately losing weight and getting fit will be very difficult. I remember feeling overwhelmed with cooking, cleaning, and taking care of my baby; much less myself. It is a daily feat to stay focused, and keep organized but it is the only way to accomplish so many important tasks in a short amount of time.

I get excited at the challenge of keeping my life in order, because the alternative feels worrisome and full of untouched potential. Trust me, our bodies can handle a great deal, but only if one continues to train and stay strong. Not to mention, your arms and back will thank you when you are holding your baby for countless hours during the day and night. Bending over to bathe a toddler is much easier when one is in the best shape possible. It is all motivation to work hard at your fitness goals, and stay positive no matter what obstacles are presented in your life!

Hormones

Hormones can cause havoc on losing the baby weight, and demolish our willingness to get motivated. Even though we may not feel great all the time, doesn't mean we cannot use the hormonal shift to our advantage. Some people call it, "Running off the crazy," or "Ridding the rage." Whatever you do, you cannot keep all of those raw emotions locked inside of your psyche and body. Keep telling yourself that working out is the only way to keep yourself and your family safe from the hormones.

In all seriousness though, Post-partum depression is a real thing; and should be taken seriously with great caution and care. I suffered from post-partum depression right after my baby was born. I felt like I was in an airplane that I knew was going to crash (that's the best metaphor I could come up with.) The feeling was terrible, and I physically hurt. It lasted for only about a week because I kept my blood flowing through working out. I forced myself to get up and get moving! I didn't want to stay on that crashing plane!

Hormones will go up and down, but there is a sudden shift right after the baby is born, and also when you wean from breastfeeding. Try not to panic, but take precautions and talk to a healthcare professional if you need to. Yoga, deep breathing meditation, stretching, and working out will help. Make sure to have a loved one available to watch the baby if post-partum depression happens. The body needs time to adjust and recover from those hormonal shifts. You're not alone in these issues, so don't be afraid to talk to family or reach out to your doctor for help.

Realizing what is happening to our bodies, will only empower you. Embrace the changes with hormones. Take it as a challenge to overcome. Giving birth to your baby was no easy feat, so losing the baby weight will not be easy either. The only kind of work that is worth doing is hard-work. It is described as "hard" for a reason, and every step of this process will be a reason to celebrate your awesomeness.

Importance of Sleep

Welcome to motherhood; let the lack of sleep begin. It is truly amazing how mothers can feed a baby every 2-3 hours, and survive on minimal sleep. Sleep really is important in many ways, but especially when losing the baby weight. In the first year, give yourself time to adapt to the new sleep routine required for your individual baby's needs. However, the more sleep you give yourself, the better you will be able to operate.

When my baby was 1 month old, I allowed my husband to feed her pumped breast milk for one feeding at night. This helped me get my eight hours of sleep. To explain: I breastfed her right before I went to sleep at 10pm, then my husband bottle-fed her my pumped breast milk at 2am, then I woke up at 6am to breastfeed her again. It really was a glorious partnership, and I was so grateful to my husband for his help.

There are many ways to get your allotted eight hours of sleep, so don't try to do this all on your own. If you are a single mom, reach out to your friends and family or someone you trust to help you get caught up on sleep. It will get easier once the baby is not feeding so often, but throughout the process sleep is very important and is imperative to weight loss.

Anytime you feel overwhelmed or behind on chores, do not beat yourself up about it. Stop what you're doing, take a deep breath or stretch, and write down 3-5 chores that need to be done that day. Most mothers know that everything changes when having a baby, but don't fret - YOU CAN AND WILL GET IT ALL DONE! Worrying about the amount of errands and chores that need to be done can cause insomnia; therefore, worrying about it does nothing but hurt you.

Each day, write down those 3-5 errands or chores that need to be done (priorities first,) and cross them off as you complete them. Please try to not lose sleep over not getting everything done. Your baby is the priority now, so strategize to get chores done, and not lose sleep about it. Writing things down when you remember is helpful; and also hanging lists up where you can see them is a must- such as the refrigerator.

The topic of Caffeine is a sensitive subject for most people, but you will sleep much more restful when eliminating it from your diet. Most people think they need their caffeine boost to function; but health care studies show that it is a very bad choice on your body. Not to mention, it will negatively affect your body's natural sleeping routine.

I decided to quit caffeine once I got pregnant, and while breastfeeding. Once the headaches and the trembling subsided, I felt so much better than before. Unfortunately, it was another chemical my body was addicted to. Caffeine can cause heart arrhythmias, and misleads the body to function in hyper drive for a limited time. It is an unnatural element to the body; therefore, should not be placed in the body.

If you are consuming Caffeine while pregnant or while breastfeeding, the baby is affected in more severe ways; because the baby's organs are not fully developed yet. Caffeine can cause the baby to develop heart troubles and/or other traumatic health issues. It is serious and should not be in your diet, much less your tiny baby's diet.

Do your own research, and don't rely on a chemical to boost your energy. Rely on natural energy boosting foods, and your body's renewable energy cycle. Doing so will help your body to regulate healthy sleep patterns; thus, providing the best sleep possible to recover and renew for top performance.

Takes Time to Recover

Whether the birth was natural, VBAC (vaginal birth after C-section), or C-section every mother needs time to recover. Therefore, there's no need to rush the process of getting back into a skimpy bikini overnight. The body is an amazing creation, and there is a reason for every step towards recovery.

Mothers gain weight during pregnancy because after delivery the body needs extra fuel to produce milk, supply energy for sleep deprivation, rearrange the body's organs back in normal position, and for many other recovery reasons. It can take about a year to drop the baby weight, naturally, and totally recover from the trauma of giving birth.

My advice is to enjoy the process of recovery, and being a new mommy! Try to be present and in the moment every day. Your baby needs you to be happy, loving, and calm. Every day is a blessing and a joy; therefore, be grateful, and don't worry the weight will come off in due time! All you have to do is stick to the plan, and enjoy your life in the meantime.

~C-section Recovery Techniques~
**If you're already passed this stage of recovery, feel free to skip ahead.

Keeping your stress level down is key with any serious surgery recovery, and a cesarean section (C-Section) is no different. However, dealing with pain can cause unwanted stress. It's normal to have pain up to two weeks after delivery, and your doctor will most likely prescribe anti-inflammatory medication, or even stronger painkillers. Everybody's pain tolerance is different, so you must do what makes you comfortable. Also, take probiotics to build back up the healthy bacteria in your gut. Antibiotics given during surgery will likely get your body's natural flora off track; which can cause diarrhea and hamper immunity.

Care for the incision as your doctor instructs. And start walking as soon as your doctor gives you the green light to do so. For me, I was standing a few hours after my C-section, because the nurses helped me and instructed me to do so. Walking will increase circulation, reduce risk of blood clots, and increase your body's healing process. All processes are sped up in the body by exercise and movement.

Eating right is also key to healing. Focus on eating anti-inflammatory foods that are high in vitamin C; such as, berries, broccoli, and kale. Vitamin C repairs tissues by supporting the production of collagen. Also, eat foods rich in omega-3 fatty acids like nuts and seeds are also inflammatory. Limit red meat- which is inflammatory. Chicken and Salmon are better choices, because they have amino acids which form proteins to repair tissues in the body.

To prevent constipation after surgery: eat fiber-rich foods, drink 100+ ounces of water, prune juice (or prunes), and ask your doctor about a stool softener. Pregnancy hormones, combined with pain killers will most likely lead to constipation. Straining can put pressure on the incision, and healing abdominal muscles- causing pain and discomfort. Also, try a toilet stool (Squatty Potty) or prop your feet on yoga blocks which will straighten the colorectal angle

Breastfeed with support by sitting up straight, and bring your baby close to you. Leaning forward will limit the amount of oxygen the body consumes (also bad for the neck as it strains it,) which will lead to fatigue and will prevent you from retaining the transverse abdominis muscles and fascia (the muscles responsible for holding your abs together.) By the way, whatever position you hold yourself (posture) is the way the body learns and adapts to. Good

23

posture leads to a stronger body- especially when healing. I enjoyed breastfeeding lying on my side because I could rest, but whatever keeps your body inline.

Things to avoid for the first 8 weeks of recovery: the abdominal binder is usually given to mothers to help with pain, but the binder will take over for the abdominal muscles- preventing the muscles from recovering. A binder will also put added pressure on pelvic organs, causing urinary incontinence. Try a graduated compression undergarment instead that will ease the pain and swelling without the other problems.

Avoid lifting anything heavy, and allow your spouse or family to help with cleaning your home. Each doctor may give a specific weight limitation on lifting, but it is usually no more than the weight of your baby. Ask for help, especially if you're in pain. Ease back into sex, and your doctor may tell you to wait for up to 8 weeks. Intercourse is more likely to be painful after a C-section delivery.

Lastly, avoid crunches because any abdominal muscle workout before the tissues are fully repaired can lead to hernia. There are 7 layers of tissue cut or disturbed during the C-section surgery, and the body needs to repair and recover fully prior to crunches. Consult your doctor about when he advises to begin an abdominal workout. Sometimes doctors will allow plank or bridge core strength training sooner than crunches, but it is always wise to ask first. Better to be safe than in pain.

~Vaginal Birth and VBAC Recovery~

There are some similarities in recovering from a natural birth compared to a C-section. Some swelling will likely occur, so use the ice-packs the nurse provides to soothe. Do not place directly onto the sensitive skin without protective fabric, and only leave on for up to 15 minutes.

Unfortunately, hemorrhoids usually happen so gently wipe with a Witch Hazel Astringent pad (Tucks) to soothe and relieve. They are also approved for use on vaginal tissue. Similar to the C-section recovery about constipation: try not to strain, and keep drinking water and/or stool softeners until it passes.

If you experienced tearing or an episiotomy, keep the wound clean and allow your body to recover before high impact exercise or movement. Even sitting on the toilet can be tortuous, so finding the most comfortable position while sitting is important. If possible, do not allow yourself to be in pain, and be sure to ask for help when you need it.

Lastly, be sure to do kegel exercises: which is the tightening of the pelvic muscles. As long as you're not in pain, work on these exercises every day. Just tighten your pelvic muscles, hold for 3 seconds, and then relax for 3 seconds. Start with 3 seconds and then add 1 second each week until you can squeeze and hold for 10 seconds.

Home Workout versus Gym

Everyone is different when finding what motivates them to workout. Some people have great, challenging routines they execute from their homes; while others enjoy going to the gym. Once everything in your life is organized and beaming with promise: adding a working out routine towards your fitness goals will only enhance the happiness!

We must find our purpose that will keep us motivated to work out. Similar to the motivation of a bride-to-be -working out to fit into her perfect wedding dress; or knowing that everything in our life will function better when we are stronger and fit. Find your purpose to why you're getting fit: your baby, looking good in skinny jeans, to feel alive and happy every day, marathon challenges, charity events, and you may have to reset your purpose frequently. Whatever drives you to work hard, is the goal and purpose for our lives.

If you decide to workout at home, be sure to have some good equipment or quality/effective routines available on DVDs for exercise. There are exercise bands, dumbbells, kettle bells, bosa ball, weight bags, and you can even use chairs for various exercises too. People can get creative at home, but just don't allow yourself to get distracted. It is easy to do when the baby cries, or your spouse asks you a question. Give yourself 30 minutes to an hour, put your music on, and focus on your routine.

Gyms can provide motivation with fitness classes and community camaraderie. Gyms are also great to separate you from home so you have time for yourself. Gyms have various exercise equipment available to you, trainers, and are usually open 24 hours a day. I personally do better at a gym, but I sometimes love working out at home too. Choose what makes you happiest and also provides the best/ effective workout.

Lastly, be sure to keep an eye on your caloric intake while working out and breastfeeding. Take care of yourself by making sure you have adequate fuel for your baby, and to compensate for your workout routine. For example, if you burn 400 calories a day from breastfeeding, and another 400 at the gym- be sure to eat the appropriate caloric intake for your Body Mass Index, plus your baby's needs. Remember, like a car, we have to provide our bodies with healthy/ adequate fuel for optimal performance!

Workout Routines

**Below are some routines to get you started, as well as suggestions on Exercise DVDs. The name of the game is: *Keep Challenging Yourself, and Get Sweaty Every Time You Workout!*

***Be sure to check with your doctor before any exercise is conducted -to make sure he gives you the green light. And if your abdominals are still in recovery, exchange sit-ups/crunches for the bridge or plank exercise or some other leg exercise until your doctor says it is okay to workout the abdominals.

I would recommend starting off slow, and gradually challenge yourself. You just had a baby, and not overdo it the first couple of weeks. Start off by doing light cardio (walking, elliptical) for 15-20 minutes 3 times a week. It is really fun to workout with your baby too! Make working out fun and enjoyable and you will want to accomplish it more often. Incorporate weight training or toning exercises only when your doctor gives you the green light, but be sure to take baby steps and work your way up. Always challenge yourself, but not go overboard. I believe in you! You got this! Workout, have fun, and Lose that Baby Weight!

30-DAY CHALLENGE

DAY 1	DAY 2	DAY 3	DAY 4	DAY 5	DAY 6	DAY 7
Pushups: 5	Pushups: 5	Pushups: 7	Pushups: 7	Pushups: 8	Pushups: 9	Pushups: REST
Squats: 50	Squats: 55	Squats: 60	Squats: REST	Squats: 70	Squats: 75	Squats: 80
Situps: 10	Situps: 15	Situps: 15	Situps: 25	Situps: 30	Situps: 35	Situps: REST
Lunges: 20	Lunges: 21	Lunges: 22	Lunges: 23	Lunges: REST	Lunges: 25	Lunges: 26
DAY 8	**DAY 9**	**DAY 10**	**DAY 11**	**DAY 12**	**DAY 13**	**DAY 14**
Pushups: 8	Pushups: 9	Pushups: 10	Pushups: 10	Pushups: 12	Pushups: 12	Pushups: REST
Squats: REST	Squats: 100	Squats: 105	Squats: 110	Squats: REST	Squats: 130	Squats: 135
Situps: 45	Situps: 45	Situps: 50	Situps: 55	Situps: 55	Situps: REST	Situps: 60
Lunges: 27	Lunges: 28	Lunges: 29	Lunges: REST	Lunges: 31	Lunges: 32	Lunges: 33
DAY 15	**DAY 16**	**DAY 17**	**DAY 18**	**DAY 19**	**DAY 20**	**DAY 21**
Pushups: 13	Pushups: 15	Pushups: 16	Pushups: 16	Pushups: 19	Pushups: 21	Pushups: REST
Squats: 140	Squats: REST	Squats: 150	Squats: 155	Squats: 160	Squats: REST	Squats: 180
Situps: 65	Situps: 65	Situps: 70	Situps: 70	Situps: 75	Situps: 75	Situps: 75
Lunges: 34	Lunges: 35	Lunges: 36	Lunges: REST	Lunges: 38	Lunges: 39	Lunges: 40
DAY 22	**DAY 23**	**DAY 24**	**DAY 25**	**DAY 26**	**DAY 27**	**DAY 28**
Pushups: 23	Pushups: 26	Pushups: 28	Pushups: 30	Pushups: 32	Pushups: 34	Pushups: 36
Squats: 185	Squats: 190	Squats: REST	Squats: 220	Squats: 225	Squats: 230	Squats: REST
Situps: REST	Situps: 80	Situps: 80	Situps: 85	Situps: 85	Situps: 90	Situps: REST
Lunges: 41	Lunges: 42	Lunges: 43	Lunges: REST	Lunges: 45	Lunges: 46	Lunges: 47
DAY 29	**DAY 30**					
Pushups: 38	Pushups: 40					
Squats: 240	Squats: 250					
Situps: 95	Situps: 100					
Lunges: 49	Lunges: 50					

30 Day Challenge to launch your weight-loss journey to success! I am a competitive person, so I enjoy challenges. Each month they change too, so keep doing these challenges if you enjoy them! Be sure to add in cardio 20-30 minutes every other day (get your heart-rate up to at least 130.)

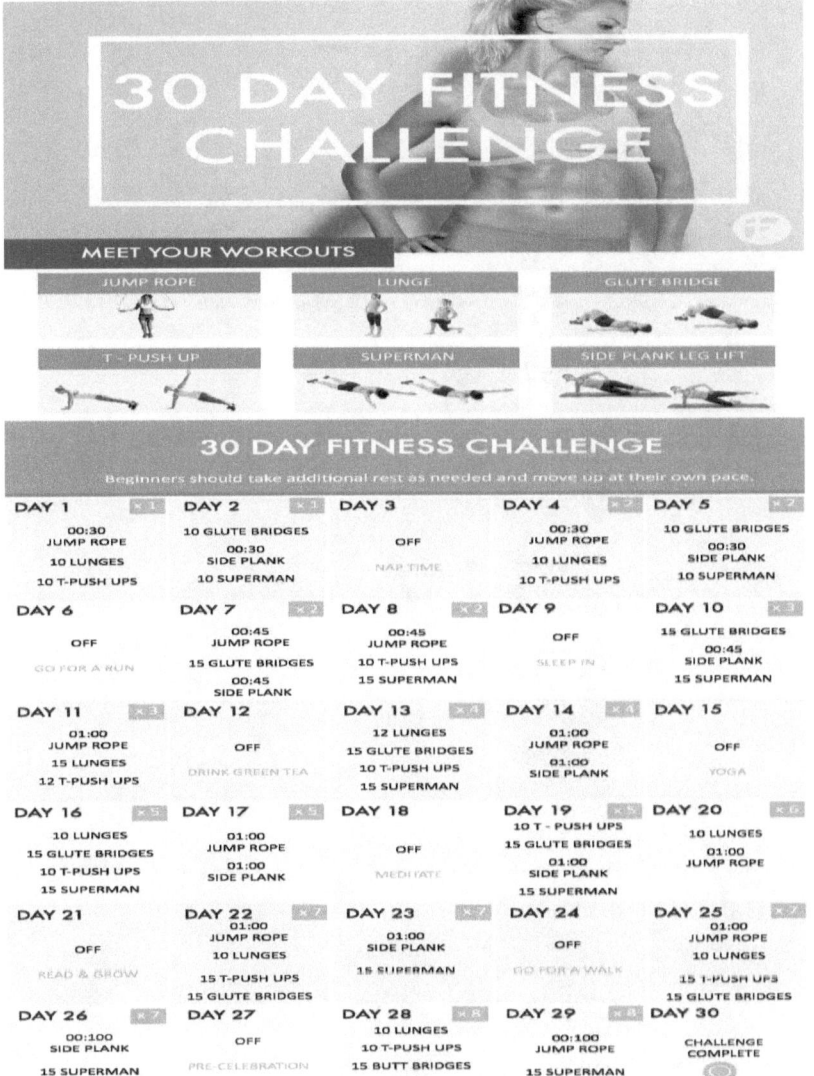

30 DAY FITNESS CHALLENGE

MEET YOUR WORKOUTS

JUMP ROPE — LUNGE — GLUTE BRIDGE

T - PUSH UP — SUPERMAN — SIDE PLANK LEG LIFT

30 DAY FITNESS CHALLENGE

Beginners should take additional rest as needed and move up at their own pace.

DAY 1 ×1
00:30 JUMP ROPE
10 LUNGES
10 T-PUSH UPS

DAY 2 ×1
10 GLUTE BRIDGES
00:30 SIDE PLANK
10 SUPERMAN

DAY 3
OFF
NAP TIME

DAY 4 ×2
00:30 JUMP ROPE
10 LUNGES
10 T-PUSH UPS

DAY 5 ×2
10 GLUTE BRIDGES
00:30 SIDE PLANK
10 SUPERMAN

DAY 6
OFF
GO FOR A RUN

DAY 7 ×2
00:45 JUMP ROPE
15 GLUTE BRIDGES
00:45 SIDE PLANK

DAY 8 ×2
00:45 JUMP ROPE
10 T-PUSH UPS
15 SUPERMAN

DAY 9
OFF
SLEEP IN

DAY 10 ×3
15 GLUTE BRIDGES
00:45 SIDE PLANK
15 SUPERMAN

DAY 11 ×3
01:00 JUMP ROPE
15 LUNGES
12 T-PUSH UPS

DAY 12
OFF
DRINK GREEN TEA

DAY 13 ×4
12 LUNGES
15 GLUTE BRIDGES
10 T-PUSH UPS
15 SUPERMAN

DAY 14 ×4
01:00 JUMP ROPE
01:00 SIDE PLANK

DAY 15
OFF
YOGA

DAY 16 ×5
10 LUNGES
15 GLUTE BRIDGES
10 T-PUSH UPS
15 SUPERMAN

DAY 17 ×5
01:00 JUMP ROPE
01:00 SIDE PLANK

DAY 18
OFF
MEDITATE

DAY 19 ×5
10 T - PUSH UPS
15 GLUTE BRIDGES
01:00 SIDE PLANK
15 SUPERMAN

DAY 20 ×6
10 LUNGES
01:00 JUMP ROPE

DAY 21
OFF
READ & GROW

DAY 22 ×7
01:00 JUMP ROPE
10 LUNGES
15 T-PUSH UPS
15 GLUTE BRIDGES

DAY 23 ×7
01:00 SIDE PLANK
15 SUPERMAN

DAY 24
OFF
GO FOR A WALK

DAY 25 ×7
01:00 JUMP ROPE
10 LUNGES
15 T-PUSH UPS
15 GLUTE BRIDGES

DAY 26 ×7
00:100 SIDE PLANK
15 SUPERMAN

DAY 27
OFF
PRE-CELEBRATION

DAY 28 ×8
10 LUNGES
10 T-PUSH UPS
15 BUTT BRIDGES
01:00 SIDE PLANK

DAY 29 ×8
00:100 JUMP ROPE
15 SUPERMAN

DAY 30
CHALLENGE COMPLETE

Fitwirr

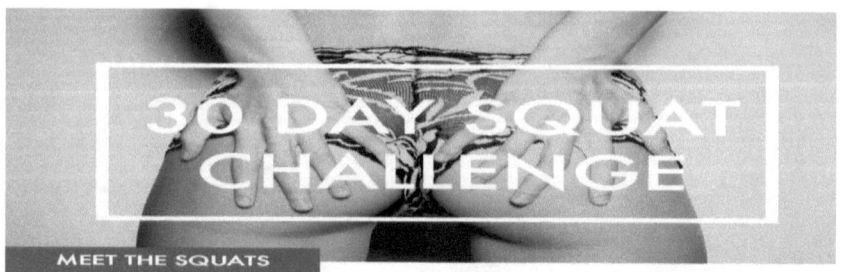

MEET THE SQUATS

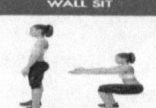
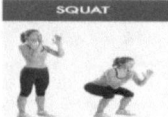
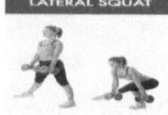
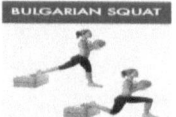

30 DAY SQUAT CHALLENGE

Free weights are optional for lateral squats and Bulgarian squats. Complete 30 days.
If you are a beginner, take additional rest and move up at your own pace.

DAY 1	DAY 2	DAY 3	DAY 4	DAY 5
00:30 WALL SIT	00:45 WALL SIT	01:00 WALL SIT	01:15 WALL SIT	OFF TAKE A NAP
DAY 6	**DAY 7**	**DAY 8**	**DAY 9**	**DAY 10**
01:30 WALL SIT	01:45 WALL SIT	30 SQUATS (10 x 3)	40 SQUATS (10 x 4)	OFF MEDITATE
DAY 11	**DAY 12**	**DAY 13**	**DAY 14**	**DAY 15**
50 SQUATS (10 x 5)	60 SQUATS (10 x 6)	70 SQUATS (10 x 7)	80 SQUATS (10 x 8)	OFF PLAY HARD
DAY 16	**DAY 17**	**DAY 18**	**DAY 19**	**DAY 20**
30 LATERAL SQUATS (10 x 3)	40 LATERAL SQUATS (10 x 4)	50 LATERAL SQUATS (10 x 5)	60 LATERAL SQUATS (10 x 6)	OFF READ & GROW
DAY 21	**DAY 22**	**DAY 23**	**DAY 24**	**DAY 25**
70 LATERAL SQUATS (10 x 7)	80 LATERAL SQUATS (10 x 8)	30 BULGARIAN SQUATS (10 x 3)	40 BULGARIAN SQUATS (10 x 4)	OFF GO FOR A WALK
DAY 26	**DAY 27**	**DAY 28**	**DAY 29**	**DAY 30**
50 BULGARIAN SQUATS (10 x 5)	60 BULGARIAN SQUATS (10 x 6)	70 BULGARIAN SQUATS (10 x 7)	80 BULGARIAN SQUATS (10 x 8)	CHALLENGE COMPLETE!

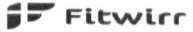

Ten Week Workout Plan

Monday

150 Jumping Jacks
50 Crunches
20 Tricep Dips
15 Squats
20 Lunges (each leg)
70 Russian Twists
20 Standing Calf Raises
5 Push-ups
30 Second Plank
10 Lunge Split Jumps

Wednesday

90 Jumping Jacks
20 Tricep Dips
10 Sit-Ups
30 Bird-Dogs
30 Second Plank
30 Squats
40 Crunches
10 Oblique Crunches (Each Side)
20 Standing Calf Raises

Friday

60 Jumping Jacks
40 Crunches
10 Sit-Ups
10 Tricep Dips
20 Side Lunges (Each Side)
15 Incline Push-Ups
10 Oblique Crunches (Each Side)
30 Butt Kickers
5 Jump Squats
15 Jack Knife Sit-Ups

Sunday

45 Jumping Jacks
15 Squats
5 Jump Squats
50 Russian Twists
30 Second Plank
10 Standing Calf Raises
5 Kneeling Push-Ups
30 Seconds Superman
10 Lunges (Each Leg)
40 Crunches

Tuesday

80 Jumping Jacks
50 Vertical Leg Crunches
20 Sit-Ups
15 Tricep Dips
20 Squats
10 Side Lunges (Each Leg)
15 Leg Lifts (Each Leg)
50 Bicycles
15 Wall Push-Ups
40 Russian Twists

Thursday

100 Jumping Jacks
25 Vertical Leg Crunches
20 Squats
20 Wall Push-Ups
50 Russian Twists
15 Second Side Plank (Each Side)
10 Lunge Split Jumps
5 Jump Squats
40 High Knees

Saturday

50 Jumping Jacks
20 Squats
100 Russian Twists
5 Kneeling Push-Ups
1 Minute Downward Dog
15 Jack Knife Sit-Ups
10 Lunges (Each Leg)
10 Side Lunges (Each Side)
20 Bird-Dogs
20 Inner Thigh Lifts (Each Leg)

Cardio (by week)

1 1 min run, 2 min walk (7x)
2 2 min run, 2 min walk (5x)
3 3 min run, 2 min walk (4x)
4 5 min run, 2 min walk (3x)
5 6 min run, 90 sec walk (3x)
6 8 min run, 90 sec walk (2x)
7 10 min run, 90 sec walk (2x)
8 12 min run, 1 min walk,
9 8 min run 15 min run,
   1 min walk, 5 min run 10 Run
10 20 minutes continuously

10 Week Workout Plan: If you like to have a routine for 10 weeks at a time, try this one!

5 Minute Kill Belly Pooch Workouts

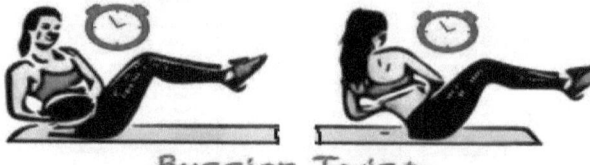

Russian Twist

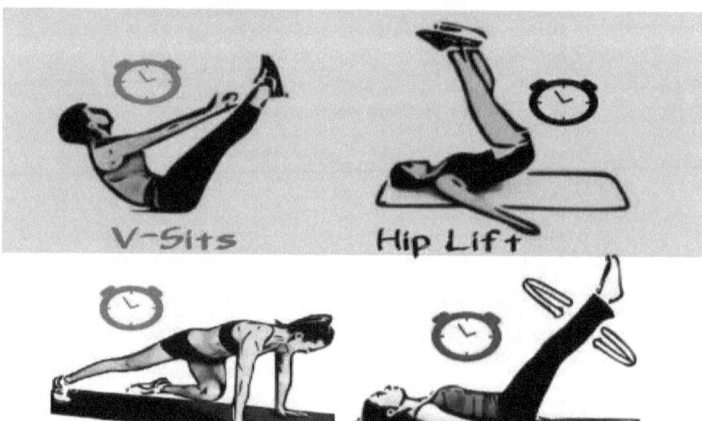

V-Sits   Hip Lift

Full plank twist   Double leg circles

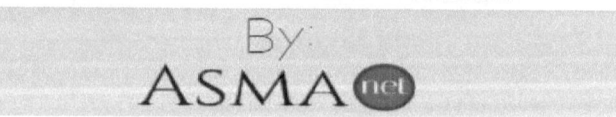

By: ASMA net

Awesome exercises to strengthen the abdominals! Incorporate this 5 minute routine into your other routines, or do this after cardio to help burn fat around the mid-section.

EXERCISE GUIDE
GYM BALL

1. Squat

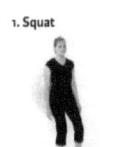 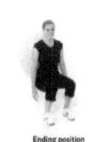

Starting position　　　　　Ending position

6. Crunch

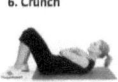 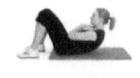

Starting position　　　　　Ending position

2. Hamstring

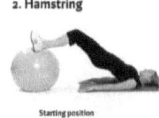 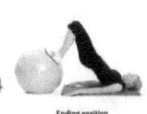

Starting position　　　　　Ending position

7. Sit-up

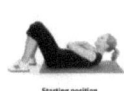 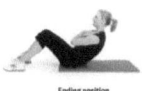

Starting position　　　　　Ending position

3. Back hyperextension

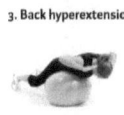 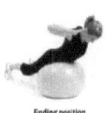

Starting position　　　　　Ending position

8. Reverse Jack-knife

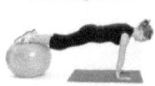 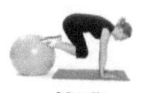

Starting position　　　　　Ending position

4. Crunch

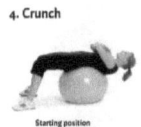 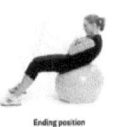

Starting position　　　　　Ending position

9. Plank rollout

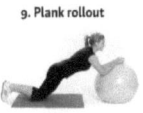 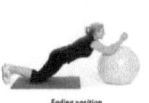

Starting position　　　　　Ending position

5. Side crunch

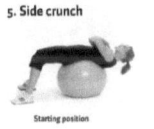 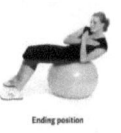

Starting position　　　　　Ending position

10. Plank

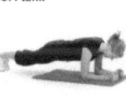

Scandic

18 MOVES
for mom & baby

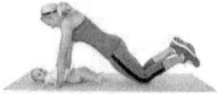

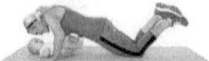

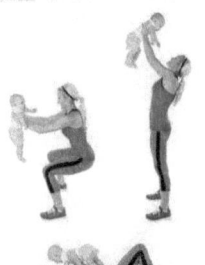

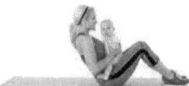

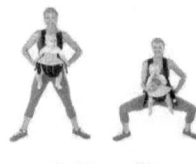

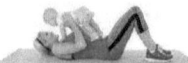

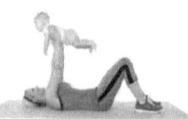

Working out with baby can be so much fun!

BABY WEARING WORKOUT

FITMOMMYFITFAMILY.COM

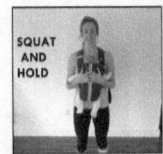
SQUAT AND HOLD

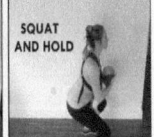
SQUAT AND HOLD

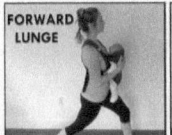
FORWARD LUNGE

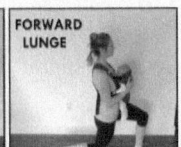
FORWARD LUNGE

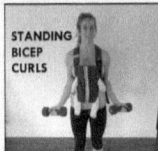
STANDING BICEP CURLS

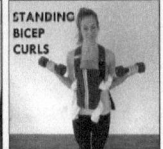
STANDING BICEP CURLS

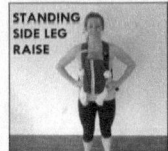
STANDING SIDE LEG RAISE

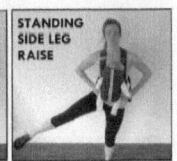
STANDING SIDE LEG RAISE

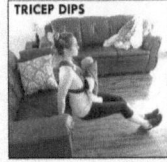
TRICEP DIPS

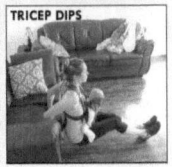
TRICEP DIPS

CIRCUIT-

COMPLETE 12 REPS OF EACH EXERCISE.

REST

REPEAT X 3

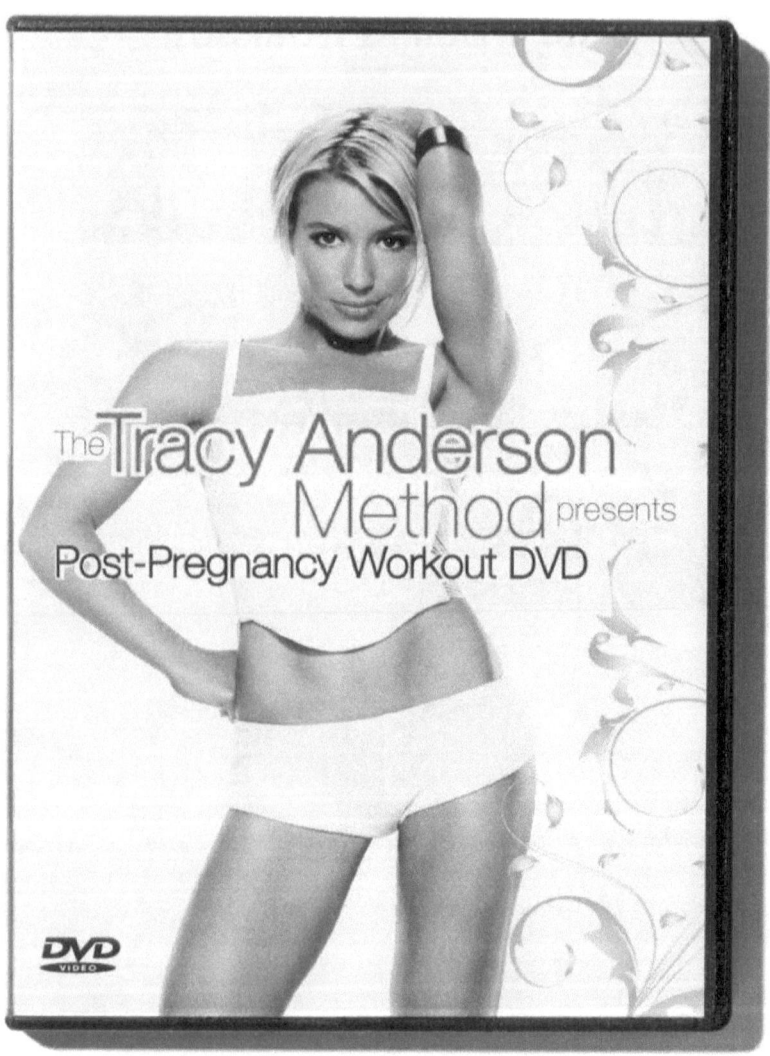

Tracy Anderson DVDs are awesome! Check them out and feel great!

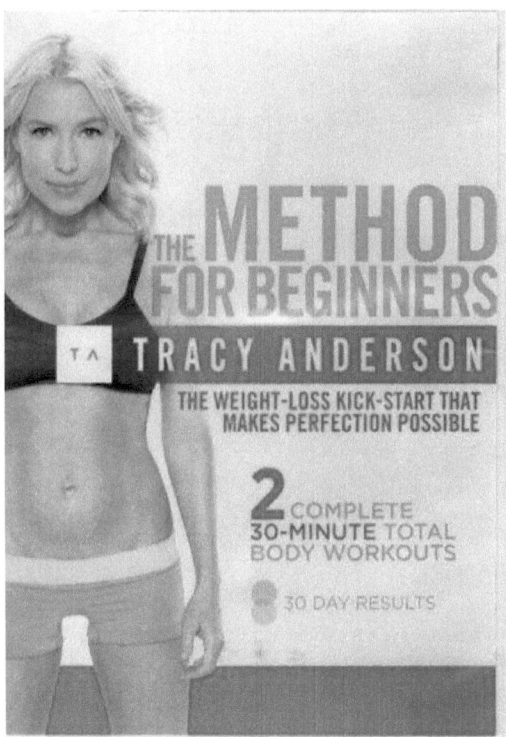

Improving Your Posture after Pregnancy and Breastfeeding

It is very important to be aware of weakened posture or what I like to call "Mommy Posture." As your pregnancy progresses, the added weight can wreak havoc on your back and your posture. But there are some easy things you can do to quickly improve your posture after pregnancy, including the use of postpartum shapewear and C-Section shapewear. Here are some tips:

Exercise 1: *Pelvic floor*
Fast and slow pelvic floor lifts not only regain bladder control of this stretched and bruised area,

but also promote circulation (which will help ease swelling) and begin to tone the deep abdominal muscles that work in conjunction with the pelvic floor.

Exercise 2: *Static tummy contractions*
Each time you feed your baby, tighten your belly and hold it for the count of ten. Repeat ten times. These are tummy flatteners.

Exercise 3: *Pelvic tilts*
Tilting your pelvis requires a gentle contraction of Rectus Abdominus, your "curl-up" muscle. This has been stretched for nine months so it needs some help shortening again! Post Six Week Check Up Moves: With an OK from your doctor, here are more toning moves you can do in about 10 minutes each day to help strengthen and recover.

Exercise 4: *Leg slides*
Building up this core strength in your tummy will also prevent hip movement during the exercise.

Exercise 5: *Shoulder squeezes*
Great for keeping your shoulders from rounding.

Exercise 6: *"Swimming"*
This is a classic Pilates-based move that engages the muscles running the length of your spine. It's very safe and simple but VERY effective. Concentrate on executing it with great control and minimal movement of your torso.

Exercise 7: *Chest/shoulder stretch*
Letting the chest and shoulders open out is vital for neck and upper back posture. This is compromised with the feeding and cuddling we do for a new baby.

Exercise 8: *Shoulder bridges*
Based on a classic Pilates move this releases tension in the spine, strengthens it and also gently stretches across the hips for a woman who has recently had a baby. A wonderful move!

Using a Foam Roller for Posture Correction
When I teach about fitness, I try to incorporate as many exercises as possible that don't require equipment. With that said, I think it's completely worth it to buy a foam roller. You can order one online or find them at any sports store (or even Target). Foam rolling helps release tension, break up pesky knots, and keep you flexible. **Please see below for photos and examples of the Foam Roll stretches for Posture Correction.

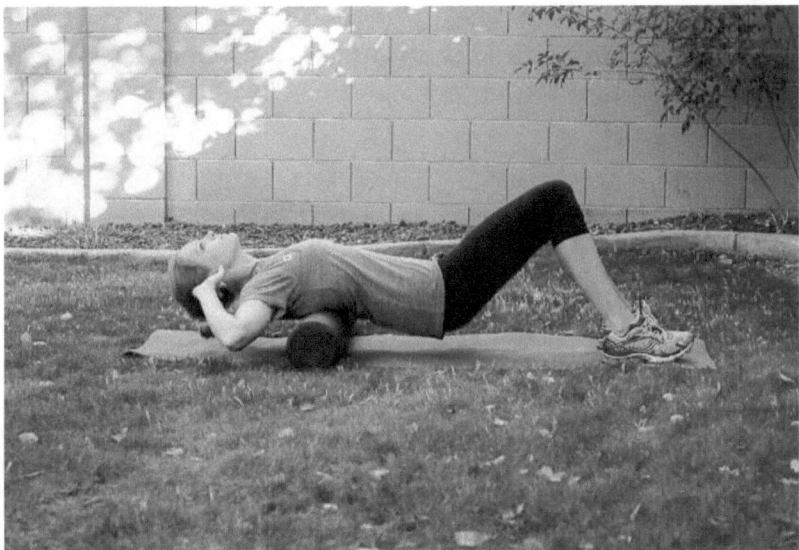

Foam Roller: Upper & Middle Back

• Lie face up with foam roller under your upper back and feet flat on the floor. Roll from the top of your back to the middle of your back in small movements with your hips elevated off the floor. If you find a spot that is particularly painful, hold for 30 seconds before moving on. **Be sure not to roll your lower back as this could cause injury.**

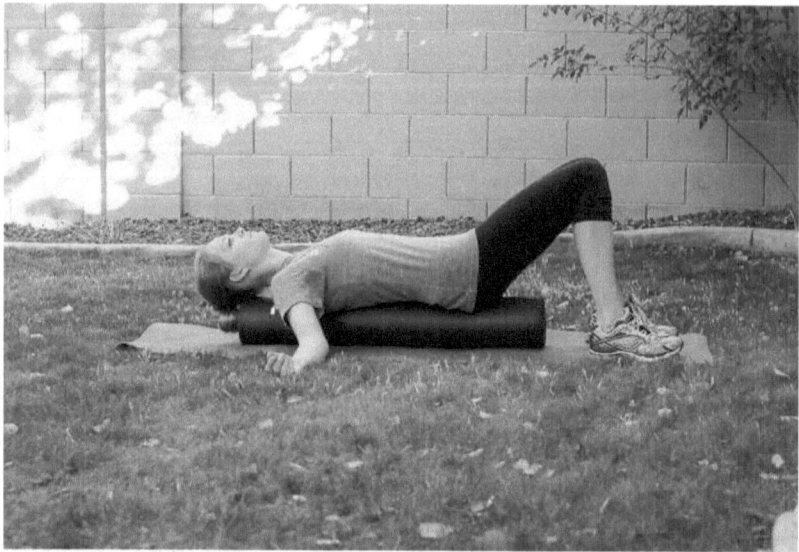

Foam Roller: Chest Stretch

• Sit on one end of the roller and then lay back. Your head should be resting on the roller and your knees should be bent with your feet flat on the floor, shoulder width apart. Drop arms out to the side and let gravity stretch the muscles of your chest and shoulders. Hold for one minute.

Repeat any and all of these exercises once a day to bring yourself back up to center.

Stretching

Stretching is so important, and can be done whenever your body is feeling tight and stiff. Be sure to warm up your muscles before stretching- by doing light cardio for 5-10 minutes. Here are some examples for full body stretching. Yoga is also a great practice for stretching and meditation. I recommend whatever makes you feel the best, but stretching is a must! **There are some stretches below to try out after Improving Your Posture section

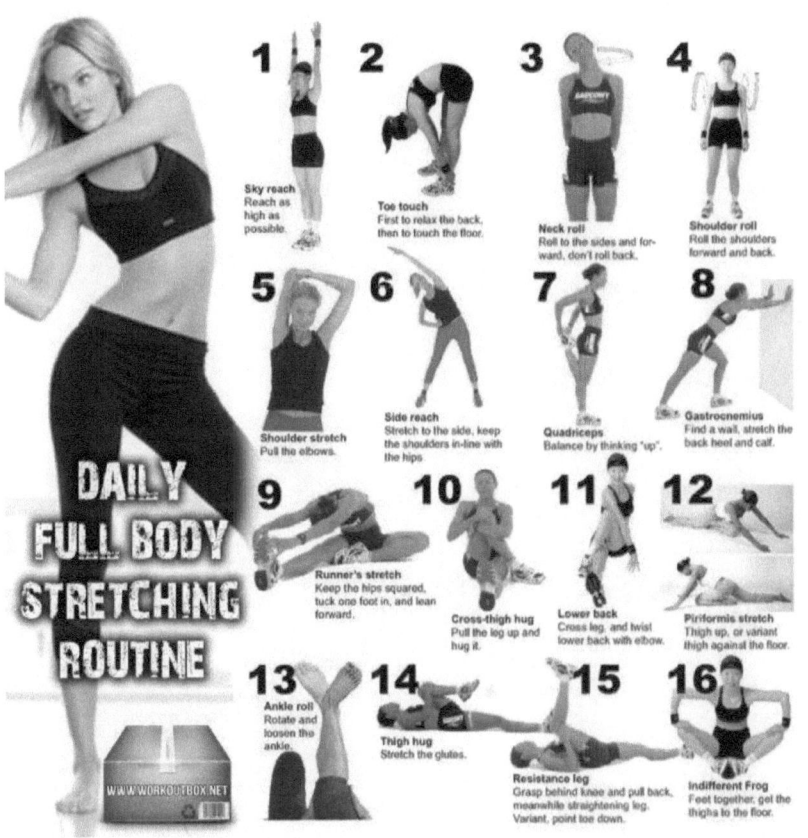

Neck and Shoulders

Back

Legs and Lower Body Stretches

Wrists

Chest, Shoulders and Fingers

Stretching Tips

- Always stretch within your comfortable limits - never to the point of pain.
- Take your time. The long sustained, mild stretch reduces unwanted muscle tension and tightness.
- If you are stretching correctly, the stretch feeling should slightly subside as you hold the stretch.
- The benefits come from regularity. Stick with it and see how you feel in a few weeks.
- Hold each stretch for at least 15 seconds and don't bounce through the stretch.
- Breathe easily and try to relax as you increase the stretch.
- Tune into your body and focus on the muscles and joints being stretched.

The highlighted exercises have been chosen by your health and fitness consultant for you given your current needs and requirements.

<u>Conclusion</u>

I hope this book will inspire you, and change your life for the better! I have learned a great deal in my travels and studies, but nothing compares to the lessons of motherhood. Seeing the World through the eyes of our children puts everything into perspective, and shows how precious every moment is. So why not be the best possible you! YOU CAN DO IT! Take these steps, and commit yourself to the transformation. I promise you will be so happy you did, and I wish you all the best! From one mother to another: Stay strong, Stay happy, and know You're Worth it! So don't ever EVER give up!

About the Author

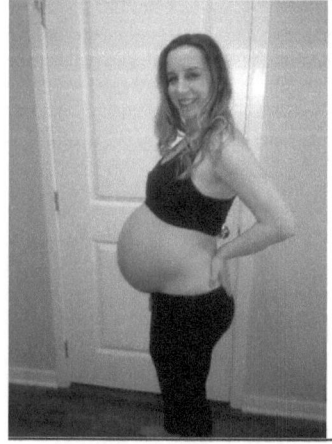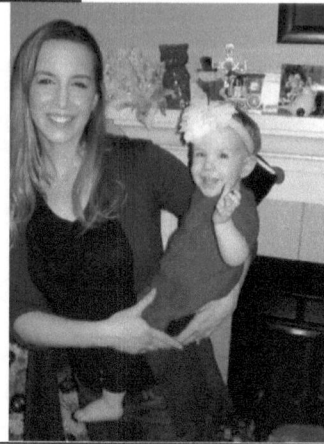

Left, Meredith Majors at 35 weeks pregnant. Right, Meredith Majors with 12month old baby Keira. Lost a total of 50 pounds in 12 months.

Meredith Majors is an English Major, originally from the Florida Panhandle. She also has certifications in Fitness and Wellness, as well as Nutrition; plus a second degree in Health. Prior to starting her family, she was a personal trainer in Los Angeles for many years. She and her husband, Chris, currently own a film production company: Savage Beast Films. Their first production is an Award-Winning Thriller titled: LAKE EERIE with World-Wide Distribution. Meredith enjoys being with her husband and daughter, and their two cats: Leonidas and Domino. She also loves going to movies, reading, writing, inspiring and helping others, being outside, cooking, and working out.

www.SavageBeastFilms.com

Losing the Baby Weight: A Quick Guide to a Fit Mind, Body, and Soul for Mothers© Author
Meredith Majors